CRUSHED HOPES

This book is excellent, excellent, excellent! Crushed Hopes is well researched and well written. It is an easy read, gripping and hard to put down. This 109-page book is packed with workable life-situation, easy-to-relate-to recovery tips and strategies. Its 24 battle-proven suggestions can help a person recover from broken dreams. Thank you, Dr. Jim Stout, for writing such a practical, inspiring book. Your books have helped so many people including me!

—Dr. Robert R. Long,
Former Executive Director, and now Chairman Emeritus, of Coalition for Christian Outreach

In this book, Rev. Dr. Jim Stout provides advice for how to bounce back from hope-crushing disillusionments. His 24 insights will guide you through how to make lemonade from lemons or wine from crushed grapes. Especially important, he provides guidelines for how to avoid rage and revenge and how to change unmet expectations into future dreams.

—Karen Mason, Ph.D., L.P.C.
Professor of Counseling and Psychology
Director of the Hamilton Counseling Program
Gordon-Conwell Theological Seminary

I feel like you wrote for me. As a young man, I never understood the appeal of a literary tragedy. Now, in my early sixties, I am successfully married for 35 years, have two wonderful sons and am a respected professional in the community. Yet, I feel some uneasiness, as if my life in some ways is a tragedy. The concept of Crushed Hopes and Unmet Expectations better defines those feeling, indicates they are normal, and gives insight into averting that potential tragedy for a happy, fulfilling life.

—Edward Rohaly

It was easy to read, very practical and helpful. I learned how to take proactive steps in overcoming disappointment. I grasped how to be flexible in order to move on from staying stuck in failed situations.

I must say the foundation of these strategies were taught to me by Leah and Jim when I was 14-18 years of age under their guidance as my youth leaders. Life comes full circle and the foundation of Christ's love for me has been the rock and hope of my letting go of all bitterness from disappointments, so they would not engulf my life. Instead, I learned to see the joy of being grateful in all things every day and the peace that brings to my soul.

—Beatriz Pando

All of us experience disappointments and unmet expectations in our daily lives. How we react and deal with them can make all the difference in how we move forward. This is the central message of "Crushed Hopes."

The book reinforced for me the importance of never forgetting the Lord is in control and has a plan for my life. It also provides simple, sage advice, and practical tools that I can use every day.

With every disappointment or unmet expectation, I have three options: give up, give in, or give it all I've got. Jim's book has been a great encouragement to me.

—John Gass

The honest openness to the painful results of crushed hopes and the choices presented exude a fountain of encouragement. I find the book such a powerful read that I am sending a copy to our daughter who has just experienced a series of crushed hopes.

—Carol Grieves

ALSO BY DR. JIM STOUT

Recovering and Rebuilding from a Severe Mental Illness

Bipolar Disorder: Rebuilding Your Life

Abandoned and Betrayed by God: Surviving a Crisis of Faith

Mental Illness and Your Marriage

9 Critical Steps to Take in a Mental Health Crisis

Boundary Setting: A Practical Guide

Boundary Setting for Clergy and Ministry Workers

A Faith That Rescues, Rebuilds, and Redeploys

Losing Control

Writings of Pain, Writings of Hope

CRUSHED HOPES

OVERCOMING UNMET EXPECTATIONS

DR. JIM STOUT

SHEPHERD
PUBLISHING

DEDICATION

This book is dedicated with gratitude to the leaders and members of the Comfort Zone Support Group, Hopes Nest Support Group, the Orange County Chapter of the Depressive and Bipolar Support Alliance, NAMI FaithNet, and my men's sharing group, The Huddle.

These special men and women have encouraged, taught, modeled, and inspired me in untold ways. I am enormously grateful for these support-group friends. Their words and actions have enabled me, time and again, to rise above my own disappointments to give positive support to people dealing with crushed hopes.

The best laid schemes o' mice and men often go astray.
—Robert Burns

CONTENTS

PREFACE

In addition to my own struggles with spoiled anticipations, I've walked alongside of countless men and women who've endured pain-filled disillusionments. If you've gone through a hope-crushing ordeal, I believe that, in spite of your current circumstances, you can weather your loss and move ahead to a happier, more fulfilling life.

The goals of this book are:

1. To show you how to avoid triggering expectations for certain people and situations.
2. To describe how to develop resiliency to hope-busted hurts that come your way.

The pages ahead will discuss how to make "crushed grapes into new wine." The coming guidelines will offer *suggested* guidelines for coping with or overcoming your unmet expectations. You will learn practical ways for when and how to raise, lower, or drop expectations for

- yourself,
- your relationships,
- difficult situations, and
- God.

For brevity, I have used the word "God," rather than always saying "Higher Power." The reader can interpret "God" whatever way he or she wishes.

Most readers prefer to read a book chronologically from start to finish. You don't have to do this. Please feel free to find your own approach. Perhaps you can begin by leafing through the parts that appeal most to you. Then later browse other topics that interest you.

Now I invite you to relax, and set aside any hurt-induced skepticism you may have developed from your letdowns. Read on to see how I and others have found help with our own crushed hopes. Discover how you, too, can overcome your own wrecked anticipations.

INTRODUCTION

Hope deferred makes the heart sick, but a longing fulfilled is a tree of life.
—Proverbs 13:12

Let's face it: everyone holds hopes for all kinds of things. Regrettably, lots of our hopeful expectations are unmet, or are permanently shattered. Often we become severely hurt due to our disappointments—with ourselves, others, organizations, or God. Persistent resentments over unfulfilled ambitions can emotionally cripple you and me, robbing us of life's joys.

If you are reading this book, you've probably suffered your share of broken dreams. If so, please know it's never too late to rebuild your hopes—or find new ones!

The Bible teaches, *"Desire realized is sweet to the soul."* [1] Yet potential disappointments lurk everywhere. The job we'd hoped for doesn't materialize; friends we counted on let us down; the romantic relationship we longed for collapses.

EVERYBODY SUFFERS DISAPPOINTMENTS

Like so many others, I've experienced plenty of disappointments—some caused by myself, some caused by insensitive people, and others caused by harmful incidents.

Although I've been through some tough times, I am exceedingly grateful that God has blessed me with his totally undeserved favor. I have an awesome wife of more than fifty-two years, two remarkable sons and their wives, five energetic grandchildren, some loyal, supportive friends, and my service and therapy dog, Thunder.

With God's help and lots of hard work, I've been fortunate to experience some successes in life: personal, athletic, academic, and professional.

Note: If you'd like to find out more details of my story, please see the About the Author section at the back of this book or visit my website at drjimstout.com.

Along with my achievements, I've also writhed with plenty of disappointments. I've suffered through countless ruined hopes—due to broken promises from others; church stresses; severe verbal, emotional, and sexual abuse by relatives; betrayals by family, friends, and colleagues; health issues; financial troubles; and other emotional upheavals.

Some of my never-ending list of smothered hopes include times when:

- As a child and teenager, I expected God to cover

my back and protect me from cruel emotional and verbal abuse, as well as years of sexual abuse by my relatives.

- I naively hoped the churches I served would appreciate my skills, caring, and sacrificial time use. I also idealistically believed that they would keep their promises on my salary and housing allowances.
- I trustingly counted on my insurance company to honor my policy and cover my hospital and medication expenses.

Although outwardly I seemed to take mistreatments well, I often imploded with inward rage at the lies or betrayals from others. Frequently, my anger often churned into resentment and bitterness.

Resentment is the number one trigger for all sorts of grave, sometimes lethal, upsets: depression, mania, panic attacks, alcohol, drug abuse, and other addictive behaviors. It probably destroys more people than anything else.

I was aware of the Bible's warning about resentment's dangers: *"See to it . . . that no bitter root grows up to cause trouble."*[2]

Regrettably, for a long time, Luke's words from the book of Acts fit me too well: *"I see that you are full of bitterness."*[3]

Finally, in the midst of my hidden resentments and count-less letdowns, I spiraled downward into a scary emotional meltdown. My inability to flex from failed hopes cost me six months of psychiatric hospitalization from November 1988 to April 1989.

Now, having gone through more than thirty years of trial and error learning, I am able to survive, even thrive, through dashed hopes. My "new normal" in dealing with expectations for myself and others is to remain flexible in my hopes and apply various recovery strategies.

After decades of hurts caused by evaporated dreams, I've finally faced up to the reality that I'll never be able to totally delete some of my painful memories. I realize that due to my past smothered hopes, I will always be emotionally vulnerable to disappointments, broken promises, and outright betrayals.

The good news is that things that used to immobilize me for months now affects me for only a day or two. Rather than marinating in resentment, anxiety, and depression, I apply a recovery strategy. Instead of losing weeks due to unhappiness, I now absorb unmet expectations like a punch in the gut and move on.

Due to old disappointments, I'm ultra-aware of my vulnerability to being hurt. I've learned how critical it is to take quick recovery action when I've suffered a shattered expectation of any kind. Because of this self-knowledge, I take proactive steps when I'm upset by a broken anticipation.

HOPEFUL EXPECTATIONS THAT DIDN'T PAN OUT

Most of us have high hopes for people, situations, organizations, companies, pets, and other things. We want our heartfelt wishes to pan out to our liking. When our desires are thwarted, we tend to get frustrated, discouraged, angry, bitter, or fearful.

Alice, a friendly, middle-aged woman, hopes to make and keep trustworthy friends. Yet recently her private confidences were breeched by some of her closest friends.

For nearly twenty-five years she'd enjoyed close, trusting relationships with four other women in her church. They'd celebrated each other's birthdays, laughed, cried, studied the Bible, prayed, shopped, and vacationed together.

Her friends promised never to tell anyone about her private information. However, last month after sharing some sensitive secrets with her "friends," Alice discovered her classified information had become common knowledge in her church.

Tragically, she found her expectation of confidentiality had been totally violated by her "trustworthy" friends.

As a result of this betrayal, Alice left her church. She grew cynical of all "religious" people, never again met with those church friends, and stopped going to that church, as well as all others.

Like Alice, we all carry hopes for other people, for ourselves, for life in general, and for God. Sadly, broken expectations can lead to serious problems if not dealt with effectively.

KEY QUESTIONS TO ASK YOURSELF

Socrates is credited with saying, "The unexamined life is not worth living." At times, excessive introspection can be confusing, even harmful. Yet self-examination can also reap constructive rewards.

Perhaps the following questions can give you a fresh look at your hopes, expectations, and dreams:

Do I have unmet expectations for myself?

- Have I set the bar of expectations for myself too low—or too high?
- Am I confident that I'll always keep my word and never violate someone's hush-hush information?
- Do I believe I will achieve most of my goals?
- Do I believe that in my life I should experience fairness, fulfillment, fun—and involve minimal suffering?

Do I have unmet hopes for other people?

- Do I hope my parents will understand and be there for me?
- Do I hope my spouse will listen to, empathize, or affirm me?
- Do I hope my children will get good grades and steer clear of drug or alcohol abuse?
- Do I hope my friends will encourage me and show care?
- Do I hope my neighbors will offer help when I need it?
- Do I hope my church leaders and fellow members will be supportive of my struggles?
- Do I hope my medical professionals (doctors,

dentists, pharmacists, nurses, and therapists) will be caring and get good results for me?

- Do I hope my store clerks and sales people will be well-mannered and helpful to me?

Do I have high hopes for touchy situations?

- Do I hope my purchased item can be readily returned with no resistance?
- Do I hope my electronic item will be repaired quickly, at no cost to me?
- Do I hope my cancelled membership will be refunded promptly, with no disagreement?
- Do I hope my insurance, phone, and TV cable companies will pay attention to my concern and be courteous, cooperative, and effective?

Do I have unmet expectations of God?

- Do I trust that God will come to my rescue when bad things happen to me?
- Do I really feel like God forgives me and genuinely loves me—in spite of my flaws?
- Do I believe God actually has confidence in me and that he wants to use my skills and experiences to make a difference in the world?

People cherish hopeful expectations for things they depend on enjoying. Unfortunately, countless individuals are badly disappointed when their hoped-for plans collapse.

However, it's never too late to re-shape an old hope—or acquire a new one! Here are twenty-four *suggested* guidelines to apply to your situation. These guides to revising your crumpled hopes—or creating new ones—may seem overwhelming or even impossible to implement. However, please don't freeze up and do nothing. You don't have to use all of the twenty-four.

As a suggestion, try reading through the guidelines in the *Table of Contents.* Then choose the ones you are drawn to.

Some recommendations may not work for you. Obviously, there's no single right way to find relief from the consequences of broken dreams. Therefore, to find healing, everyone must find his or her own path through shattered expectations.

As you read the pages ahead, please apply the saying of *Alcoholics Anonymous:* "Take what works and leave the rest."

I

LET GO OF UNMET EXPECTATIONS

ACCEPT THE REALITY OF YOUR LOST HOPES

We must let go of the life we have planned, so as to accept the one that is waiting for us.
—Joseph Campbell

Sooner or later, coming to terms with an irreversible loss is essential. It helps to start by evaluating your deficit with the cold, hard facts of your situation. Look at the reality of "what actually *is*," apart from your aspirations. Are you rationalizing your hopes? Discuss your wished-for situation with wise friends. Ask them if your hope is truly realistic. Be open to hearing their feedback.

The unpleasant fact is that some circumstances and people will *never* change. As much as you hope, pray, manipulate, or plead, it is sobering to accept that an amputated limb will never grow back, a job will not return, a lover will not respond with like affections.

Are you worn out from your attempts to rescue your vaporized hope? You may have tried everything you knew to restore your ravaged expectancy, again and again, yet with no positive results.

Einstein was familiar with fruitless attempts to fix a broken situation. He is often quoted defining insanity as, "Doing the same thing over and over, each time expecting different results."

If you are trying your best to accept the pain of a vanished dream, perhaps you might pray something like this:

> Lord, please give me the courage to give up my compulsion to change people and situations to fit *my* expectations. Help me to see that it is *I* who needs to be changed, not others.

In my case, I had to release what *was*, so that I could come to grips with what *is now*. I believe this attitude switch has strengthened me to pursue what *will be*.

Following my second set of two total knee replacement surgeries, I had to comprehend that some of my sports expectations were wiped out—probably forever. My hopes for continuing my favorite sports were history. No more jogging or running. No more playing racquetball and handball. No more regular bicycling—my knees wouldn't bend enough. No more trudging through heavy woods on hunts for deer or wild boars. No more wading in streams on fishing trips.

I mourned these losses as terrible, often absorbed with feeling sorry for myself, resentment, and depressive dips.

The heart-wrenching reality was that my fun-filled sports and exercise routines were simply *gone*—forever. I had to give up those dreams, and trust God to show me *alternative* hopes that I would find acceptable.

For a while, I was afraid to let go of what was enjoyable in order to try something new. There was a sense of security in the familiar. I had to learn new ways to cope with my missed wishes. In essence, I needed to accept my losses and move on.

Finally, after processing my new, unwanted reality, I modified my hoped-for prospects. I turned to new exercises like walking on level ground and in the swimming pool, recumbent bicycling, flat-land hunting, and lake fishing.

Although I'm a recovering bulimic and not an alcoholic, I occasionally attend AA and other 12-step meetings for the support and recovery tips I receive. I've found that the common AA meeting themes of recovery tips for pain, resentment, and fear apply to many life issues beyond alcohol addiction.

The "big book," *Alcoholics Anonymous*, helped me to understand that when I was disturbed, it was because I found some person, place, thing, or situation was unacceptable to me. I had to face the fact that there would be no serenity for me until I *accepted* that circumstances were exactly the way they were supposed to be at that moment.

Finally, I really understood that until I accepted life completely on its terms along with its ruined hopes, I couldn't be happy. I needed to focus not so much on what needed to be changed in the world but on what needed to be changed in my attitudes.

Acceptance was the key for me. In time, I finally realized that I didn't have to like my losses, but I did need to acknowledge their *reality*. What a life-changing difference it has made in my outlook on disappointments.

QUESTIONS TO PONDER:

- Have you really come to terms with your demolished hopes?
- What new hope(s) can you find?

COUNT THE COST OF PURSUING YOUR FADING DREAM—FOR YOU AND OTHERS

Don't be too scared to calculate risks.
—Sunday Adelaja

Sometimes, it's worth taking risks. When things work out well the rewards are awesome, but when things fail, the downside can be disastrous.

I recommend making a written list of the *undesirable* costs of rehashing your failed hope—the time spent obsessing on your loss, money lost on squandered efforts, or your tainted relationships with others.

This means making a cost-benefit analysis of your lost hopes. Are you minimizing the negative effects of continuing to pursue your evaporated expectation? Is it worth hanging on to your destructive feelings and the derailed lifestyle you now have over your crushed hope?

When I started publishing again, I had the ambitious plan to finish all of my books within one year. Looking back, it was overly idealistic for me to press on with my self-imposed deadline of publishing thirteen books in twelve months! I would have forfeited too much. I would have suffered, as would my wife, family, friends, and my overall emotional and physical health.

Calculating those potential time and energy sacrifices proved to be a wise decision. I'm grateful for having made it and for what's come from it. Taking a hard look at the collateral damages from *continuing* to rescue my dream forced me see the negative effects I was imposing on myself and others.

Counting the costs of retrieving my disappeared hope proved to be a wake-up call for me. The costs were too great. I was compelled to modify my hopes in order to match what was most important to me and my true priorities.

QUESTIONS TO PONDER:

- What are the negative consequences to you and others of continuing to revive your hope?
- What are the positives for you and others of releasing your deflated hope and moving on?

3

LET GO OF YOUR ASPIRATIONS FOR YOURSELF, OTHER PEOPLE, OR SITUATIONS

Some people believe holding on and hanging in there are signs of great strength. However, there are times when it takes much more strength to know when to let go.
—Ann Landers

The most important lesson I and other lost-hope over-comers have learned for surviving our gone-astray hopes is to make a clear choice to lower or completely let go of our hoped-for desires.

Here are two suggestions from fellow survivors of crushed hopes:

First, be prepared in case your hopes for yourself, people, or situations don't turn out as you had hoped. Mentally protect yourself from collapsed hopes by expecting little or nothing. Then you'll never get let down. Maybe you'll be pleasantly surprised at times.

An unknown philosopher writes, "Blessed is he who expects nothing, for he shall never be disappointed."

One battler of destroyed hopes shares, "If you expect nothing from anybody, you'll never be disappointed."

Research shows that expecting maximum fun on a holiday often leads to big disappointments. People who make elaborate plans and believe they'll enjoy their time to the fullest were the most dissatisfied afterward.

When you are trapped in thoughts about what should be coming to you, you'll be surrounded by unrelenting anxiety. This worry isn't conducive to your emotional serenity.

When you stop expecting people to be perfect, you can like them for who they are.

It's imperative to accept things *as they are*, not *as you want them to be*. Likewise, it is critical to either modify or let go of your tightly held plans.

Inner peace is possible only when you adjust or let go of your ambitions for yourself or others. Then turn them over to the Creator of the Universe who created you and knows what's best for you.

This means that it's usually necessary to surrender—over and over—your hoped-for results to God.

Second, to sidestep huge disappointments, try applying these mottos for dealing with broken expectations and potentially hope-deflating situations:

- Limited expectations mean limited disappointments.

- Expect nothing and appreciate everything.

Portia Nelson was a popular American singer, songwriter, actress, and author. Her life was a remarkable example of letting go of one hope and finding another.

Nelson's renowned singing and acting career was cut short by several life-threatening bouts with breast, throat, and tongue cancers.

Due to these dream-depriving obstacles, she substituted two other aspirations: writing and composing. As a result of Portia Nelson's courageous exchange of her robust singing career, her writing and composing have inspired countless people.

A case in point is her book of writings *There's a Hole in My Sidewalk: The Romance of Self-Discovery*. It contains her legendary poem, *Autobiography in Five Short Chapters*, which is used as a vital part of recovery literature for 12-step groups.

Last year I found Dr. Henry Cloud's book, *Necessary Endings*, to be an enormous help in dealing with my expectations. It gave advice on ending certain relationships and projects: whether or not to hang onto these, or when and how to end certain hopes related to my consulting, counseling, and relationships. I've recommended it to various physician friends, business leaders, and others. I wish I had read it long ago.

QUESTIONS TO PONDER:

- Are you at a fork in the road on deciding whether to lower or completely let go of your expectations?
- What resources can you use in your decision making?

4

LET GO OF YOUR HURT, ANGER, AND DESIRE FOR REVENGE

Hate is like acid. It can damage the vessel in which it is stored as well as destroy the object on which it is poured.
—Ann Landers

It will help to remind yourself that recovering from the death of a dream is a *process*. No matter how spiritual you may be, there is no quick fix. Chris Gardner opined, "Baby steps count, too, as long as you're moving forward."

Fellow flattened-dream survivors and I suggest making conscious decisions to trust again and to live with a heart open to new possibilities. Forgiveness starts with a decision, but it is not an instant, one-time deal. Even for the most spiritual person, forgiving, letting go and moving on is a *process* that can take months or years. Be patient with your inflamed feelings. It will take time to heal. So keep trying to forgive, and move ahead with your life.

The Bible discourages revenge, saying, *"Do not say, I'll pay you back for this wrong! Wait for the Lord, and he will deliver you."* [1]

Author Idowu Koyenikan writes, "But if you forgive someone for something they did to you, it doesn't mean you agree with what they did or believe it was right. Forgiving that person means you have chosen not to dwell on the matter anymore; you have moved on with your life."

I like Carrie Fisher's insights into revenge: "Revenge is like drinking poison and waiting for the other person to die."

Whenever your anger surfaces, it will be helpful to write about your thoughts, then talk about your distresses with both a reliable friend and God.

Denise, a loyal and effective employee of a major commercial airline, looked forward with anticipation to retiring from her airline position with full pension benefits.

Suddenly, as a "cost-saving strategy" for the company, she and numerous others were laid off. This unexpected action happened just thirty days before her full pension would have kicked in. She was both hurt and enraged.

Tragically, Denise couldn't and wouldn't let go of her anger. She refused to release her desire to take some kind of revenge. As a result of her "unfair" treatment, she grew more and more bitter. In less than a year, her disillusionment with the company precipitated her into heavy drinking and a lethal heart attack.

Oh, how I identify with Denise. Some twenty years ago at a 12-step meeting, I shared my ongoing anger over my "Christian" insurance company's duplicity on my policy coverage. A female member of the group shared with me some pages on resolving resentment from *Alcoholics Anonymous (The Big Book).*

As I began to apply them, those words gradually dissipated my intense anger. I've gone back to those statements time and again to get help with other anger matters. I commend to you pages 64–67 from the book, *Alcoholics Anonymous (The Big Book).*

Victims of wounds from unrealized hopes caution those who try to forgive too hastily in order to make peace and resume "normal" relations.

Picture yourself hammering a large nail into a piece of wood. Then, visualize pulling the nail out. With a quick yank, it's out. But the puncture hole in the wood remains. You can cover it up with filler, but the well-disguised, painted-over cavity will always be there.

Likewise, when you forgive someone, the memory of the offense will grow fainter in time, but the scar will always remain, and remembrance of the affront will never totally go away.

As you make efforts to forgive, beware of false reassurances by your promise-breaker. Forgive, but don't naively forget. Despite any promises to reform, avoid trusting the offending person or organization until a positive track record has been established. If you trust too soon, you are vulnerable for another, perhaps far worse, wounding.

QUESTIONS TO PONDER:

- What steps have you taken to forgive and move on?
- Are you willing to take a few minutes to read a few pages from *Alcoholics Anonymous*?
- Are you open to trying a 12-step meeting of your choice?

5

DON'T SECRETLY CLING TO YOUR EXPECTATIONS

Ain't no shame in holding on to grief . . . as long as you make room for other things too.
—Bubbles from "The Wire"

Despite their mental acceptance of a loss, some people, deep down, still cling to the hope that their situation will change; God will intervene with answered prayers, or their spouse will be transformed, or their boss will relent.

There are instances when a loss is so great that there is no possible *Plan B*. There is no acceptable "cavalry horse" that can substitute for your nostalgic longing, your deflated dream, or your forever-lost hope. It simply is what it is: a huge, aching loss that leaves you numb and sad beyond words.

Sometimes to avoid the unending anguish that can eventually poison your relationships, it's necessary to accept the heartbreaking reality that there will be no *Plan B* for your extinguished hope and that you need to move on.

Finally resigning yourself to the reality of your unrecoverable dream is sobering beyond words. It's like you are left standing alone at the pier, watching your hope sail away with all your unmet expectations.

Ditching efforts to return to your dearly loved sport is like watching a sports event knowing your athletic injuries will forever prevent you from participating again.

What can you do if you are in this lonely, agonizing, seemingly endless state where no other dream can replace your terrible loss? No new or revised dream is possible, satisfactory, tolerable, or good enough. You are simply stuck in a forlorn desert with your permanently snuffed-out possibilities.

Eventually though, it will be necessary to make a hard choice. You will decide to accept your new normal, or you will choose to harden yourself against more pain by living the rest of your life in self-imposed misery, immersed in self-made, regret, resentment, or cynicism at yourself, others, or God.

The bottom line is that you *can* find release from your long-endured lost hope—not easily, but doable. While it may seem overly simplified, we crushed hopers have found that when no acceptable *Plan B* dream was possible for us, we had to:

- grieve our losses,

- accept that "It is what it is. Accept it and move on, shifting gears as best we could," and
- ask God for ongoing help and guidance.

In doing so, we trusted that God would help and guide us in our shaky new steps out of our barren deserts.

We found great encouragement from Scripture promises like:

> Forget the former things; do not dwell on the past. See, I am doing a new thing! Now it springs up; do you not perceive it? I am making a way in the wilderness and streams in the wasteland. The wild animals honor me, the jackals and the owls, because I provide water in the wilderness and streams in the wasteland, to give drink to my people.

—Isaiah 43:18–20

Most hopes can be replaced by another, but some are irreplaceable, so it's both wise and prudent to think ahead to the possibility that your current hope may not work. This will necessitate making some kind of backup strategy or standby substitute.

QUESTIONS TO PONDER:

- What are your forever-gone hope(s)?
- What areas in your life are you trying to satisfy with unrewarding things?
- How can you find true fulfillment in God alone?

II

DEVELOP REALISTIC EXPECTATIONS

6

TAKE A MENTAL INVENTORY OF
YOUR LETDOWNS

Ponder the path of your feet . . .
—Proverbs 4:26

Describe your hoped-for expectation by putting it into words. Then share both your crushed hope and your reactions with a friend.

As you take your inventory, here are a few questions to ask yourself. They may shed light on some of the side-effects from your unfulfilled dreams. Your reactions may be a clue that you are reacting adversely to your loss.

- Have I been feeling anxious, depressed, resentful, numb, or ashamed?
- Am I avoiding certain people or situations?
- Am I grappling with a compulsive, self-sabotaging behavior such as overwork or eating problems, or

an addiction like alcohol, drugs, sex, gambling, or something else?

To combat my own mood swings and addictive nature, I write about my thinking patterns and emotional responses. Then I share them with several close friends and my therapist. Their feedback is validating, encouraging, and informative.

SUGGESTED STEPS TO TAKE:

- Take a few minutes to jot down your thoughts and feelings about recent disappointments.
- Share them with a trusted person.

7

IF YOU OFTEN HAVE UNREALISTIC EXPECTATIONS, LOWER YOUR EXPECTATION BAR

Disappointments are inevitable; discouragement is a choice.
—Dr. Charles Stanley

The hopes of some folks are oftentimes super lofty. Their apple pie in the sky expectations are caused by having an unrealistic assessment of themselves, others, or the situations they're in. They hold on to impractical fantasies for the perfect vacation, the ideal spouse, the talented child, or the ever-loyal friend.

In his book, *A Million Miles in a Thousand Years*, Donald Miller observes that *lower* expectations actually lead to more overall happiness. Around 2009, *60 Minutes* featured a story based on a study by a British university that ranked the happiest countries in the world, excluding health and financial position. Denmark topped the list while America was near the bottom.

Why did the Danes have such contentment? Mainly because they had *low* expectations. Their culture promoted looking at life realistically, without expecting *things* to fulfill their relationships or eliminate all their problems.

As a result of this happiness-contentment report, Miller shares that he dropped all expectations that *anything* or *anyone* will ever be perfect.

When he ceased mentally demanding that people be flawless, he was able to like them in spite of their faults. Because he stopped expecting God to solve all his problems, he discovered how much more he enjoyed talking with God. Since he stopped searching for possessions and achievements to give him lasting satisfaction, he started to enjoy what he had.

In my case, my determined hope was to complete the thirteen books I'd been working on for the past fourteen years. Unfortunately, life got in the way and I still have seven nearly completed manuscripts to finish. Although I had done my due diligence on all possible writing hindrances, several unexpected health issues and other obstacles blocked my progress.

I had to lower, or at times revise, my hopes into more manageable chunks. This has been a humbling experience for my Type-A, ambitious focus. Lowering my "expectation bar" has eliminated several deadline pressures. It has also provided time to do better research, achieve more quality writing, and spend more time with my family and hobbies.

QUESTIONS TO PONDER:

- Are you willing to lower your hopes?
- If so, what will your changed expectations look like?

8

IN CERTAIN CASES, TRY RAISING YOUR EXPECTATION BAR

The man who does not value himself, cannot value anything or anyone.
—John Joseph Powell

Most folks with low self-esteem think poorly of their own abilities and future. Maybe you struggle with shaky self-confidence. If so, how about taking some new steps to *boost* your expectations—for yourself, certain people, or specific situations?

Poor self-image can have many causes. It may result from a dysfunctional family, a disability, or the destructive words or actions of others. Countless individuals develop an inferiority complex that demolishes their self-assurance.

Too often a person's sense of self-worth is shredded by being lied to, belittled, or betrayed by an abusive teacher, relative, friend, coach, coworker, or boss. These can wound self-respect to the point where it's difficult to generate anything other than minimal or no hope for yourself, others, life, or God.

How do you jack up your excessively low expectations, especially when your dreams are so limited and perhaps self-defeating?

The author Ayn Rand's words offer a concrete way to rebuild a trauma-damaged self-value for the person who's been victimized:

> It is an absolute human certainty that no one can know his own beauty or perceive a sense of his own worth until it has been reflected back to him in the mirror of another loving, caring human being.

The father of one of my high school classmates constantly demeaned him with cutting words like, "You're a miserable failure, a lifetime loser. You'll never amount to anything."

His father also continually made and broke promises such as, "I'll buy you a new bicycle. I'll buy you your first car. I'll be at your graduation."

The results of his father's ongoing mistreatment? To this day, my fifty-two-year-old friend holds little trust in the words of anyone. His self-loathing shadows him everywhere. Due to his father's negative predictions, he can barely play golf, a sport he loves, without playing a miserable round. He's beaten every time he steps up to hit the ball, and it goes the same way for anything he attempts.

My friend's life is marked by ever-present depression because he has no hope that his father's "failure curse" will ever go away.

Even though my colleague is exceptionally talented, he sees only negative possibilities for himself, his wife, his kids, his friends, his work—even his golf game and other hobbies.

He doesn't even try to imagine that he can succeed at anything. He has no hope or possibilities that his life will ever be different. For him, life is one never-ending, resent-ment-filled pity party.

How life-changing it would be if he could grab onto Eleanor Roosevelt words, "No one can make you feel infe-rior without your consent."

My friend must see that he has options for reacting to his devastating background. He can choose to live as a help-less, hopeless person, fully disapproving of himself and mistrusting everyone.

Or he can take practical steps to heal his impaired psyche. He can opt to get help for changing his self-destructive thinking. Using recovery tools and tactics, he can ferret out a new hope for himself.

No longer will he be chained to a pre-written script for his life. He can break the verbal abuse that has chained him for so long.

The good news is my friend has processed most of his crippled self-view. It's taken a long time, but he's utilized talk therapy and read voraciously on self-image improvement. Today he looks at himself, people, and life from a whole new perspective.

If you are shackled by low self-esteem, you, too, can free yourself from others' words and behaviors that have stolen your happiness. Like my friend, you really can give yourself a self-image makeover by rebuilding your self-esteem and developing a more optimistic outlook on yourself, life, people, and God.

Maybe your self-image rehabbing prayer could be something like, "God, please give me courage to hope for the best in myself, others, and you. Help me to trust you. Please lead me to resources that will benefit me."

Here are a few suggestions from many self-image battlers, including me, who have found healing and new confidence. Make every effort to:

- receive wise counseling from a caring therapist;
- surround yourself with positive, affirming friends;
- read self-help books on self-image issues by authors like Jack Canfield, Robert Schuller, Norman Vincent Peale, James Dobson, Cecil Osborne, Zig Zigler, Anthony Robbins, or others;
- ask God for help and guidance;
- reach out in some way to encourage others or help those who can't repay you in any way; and
- accomplish a few personal or professional tasks *every* day.

THOUGHTS TO PONDER:

- You can become a new you—with breathtaking possibilities you never imagined. At last, you can start to imagine big by picturing how God can use your past hurts along with your unique skills to impact people and the environment!
- Verbal or emotional abuse do not have to be your predestined life script. You can break free from those sick, false pronouncements. You can raise your expectations for yourself, others, and God. You can learn to trust again. Begin visualizing the "new you" that is being formed: a brave, talented, caring, serving person. Remind yourself often that your unique personality, special skills and experiences are desperately needed by the world.
- Be patient with yourself, people, and life. The new you will take time. Keep in mind that it's progress, not perfection, that counts.

9

GO WITH THE SOLUTION THAT WORKS, NOT ONE THAT SHOULD WORK

Finding solutions, ones that last and produce good results, requires guts and care.
—Henry Rollins

It's important to find what best produces your desired result. A workable answer will protect you from repeated hope-crushing defeats. Whenever possible, reduce your exposure to toxic situations, and keep totally away from potential harm.

Maybe your frustration over your anticipated solution is due to the recurring failure from your mechanic, your insurance company, your utility company, your cell phone carrier, or something else.

The following persons experienced one shattered hope after another. Can you relate to their hopes of finding an effective solution to their problems?

Marilyn hoped this was *the* medication to solve her health issue. Yet she was plagued by its unbearable side effects. Still, her doctor stubbornly refused to change her medication, and so she meekly accepted his insistence that she remain on it. She gave up hope in her medication and resigned herself to tolerating her daily vomiting from it.

Jeff hoped for fun workouts in his fitness club, but half the showers in the men's locker room didn't work. He wore himself out requesting repairs. His complaints got nowhere, even after five months of asking for changes. Exasperated, he terminated his membership and joined a different gym.

Helen had high hopes of enjoying her new computer and what it could do for her. Then she encountered one electronic glitch after another. Each time she took it to the computer store, only to have a technician tell her the problem was a hardware or software matter. When she returned home, she discovered the very same trouble occurred again and again. Exasperated that after several attempts the technicians couldn't fix her problem, she sold her computer and bought a different brand.

Here are a few steps you might consider taking when you're not getting your issue resolved. First, let your provider know of your dissatisfaction. Explain that you want the problem fixed as soon as possible. Set a *specific* time limit for a positive resolution for when it must be corrected.

Second, if your problem isn't corrected within your deadline, take action to make changes:

- go to the top of the management chain (don't waste any more time with technicians or sales reps —directly contact supervisors, general managers, boards of directors, or mass media);
- ask for a full refund;
- cancel your order;
- report the poor work to appropriate authorities; or
- change to another carrier, doctor, health club, or computer firm.

QUESTIONS TO PONDER:

- Has your issue been satisfactorily remedied by your deadline? If not, perhaps it's time for you to go another route.
- What different route can you choose?

10

REVISE YOUR PAST GOALS OR SET NEW ONES

Progress always involves risks. You can't steal second base and keep your foot on first."
—Frederick Wilcox

It's not a question of *if* your hopes, dreams, or plans don't turn out as you hope. It's *when* they go amiss. When your expectations go amiss, what can you do?

Give up? Kick your life into neutral gear and do nothing but exist, waiting for your hopes to come back?

Or do you set new goals?

Noah, a trim sixty-year-old former college athlete shuffled out of his doctor's office in shock. He'd just been told he had advanced Alzheimer's disease.

This unexpected medical prognosis meant his expectations for the coming years were deleted. No more traveling with his wife. No more trips with his children and grandchildren. No more jogging, playing racquetball, or skiing.

Noah holed up in his house for the next four months, refusing to go anywhere or be with anyone other than his wife. Unable to see ways of altering his long-held dreams or developing new plans, his mental capacities rapidly diminished. He died a year later.

There's a saying by the old U. S. Cavalry that goes something like, "If your horse dies, find another horse, saddle up, and ride on."

If your hoped-for expectation dies, work at discovering a new hope and move ahead. This takes courage, resolve, and a willingness to make educated gambles. Former Harvard University President, J. B. Conant, urged people to take more risks: "Behold the turtle—he makes progress only when he sticks his neck out."

An anonymous author challenges those of us who are dealing with ceasing-to-exist dreams to make a choice: "Live the rest of your life as a memorial service, or you can put it away and get on with it."

John Greenleaf Whittier penned these sorrowful words, describing those who neglect goal-setting, planning, and follow-through:

> For of all the works of tongue
>   and pen,
> The saddest of these: It might have
>   been!

Yes, "moving on" is hard. It's complicated. And messy. Yet a good starting place is to *revise* your hopes, expectations, goals, and plans, or set new ones. In time, as you emerge from grieving over your ruined possibility, you'll be free to reinvest your energies in a different hoped-for dream that could come true.

The Bible gives God's reassurance: *"For I know the plans I have for you . . . plans to prosper you and not harm you, plans to give you hope and a future."*[1]

I've always enjoyed reading books on leadership, goal setting, overcoming adversity, suffering, and similar topics. My association with strong leaders over the years and reading the writings of various authors have been heavy-duty fortifiers as I passed through diverse disappointments.

One of the recent inspirational books I've enjoyed has been John Mason's *Don't Wait for Your Ship to Come In—Swim Out to Meet It!* His paperback is filled with "bite-sized inspirational quotes to help you achieve your dreams."

However, it is wise to carry your hoped-for dream *loosely*. Be careful not to let your expectation morph into an entitlement to be met. Allow your new hope to be a firm *guideline*, rather than an entitled, unbreakable expectation. Allow your goals to bend. As the saying goes: "If you don't learn to flex a little, you'll soon be bent out of shape."

Please don't be afraid to dream again, to chart a new course, or to undertake a risky adventure. Just thinking about fresh possibilities can strengthen you if you are overwhelmed by your crushed hopes. It's worth it to start creating in your own mind a different expectation goal.

QUESTIONS TO PONDER:

- What new or revised possibilities can replace your collapsed hopes?
- Have you written down deadlines and measurable ways to assess your progress?
- With whom can you share your new plans?

11

PLAN AHEAD FOR FUTURE, UNMET EXPECTATIONS

Failing to plan is planning to fail.
—Ben Franklin

The Bible states, *"The wisdom of the prudent is to give thought to their ways, but the folly of fools is deception. . . . The prudent see danger and take refuge, but the simple keep going and pay the penalty."* [1]

The old adage is certainly true: "If you aim at nothing, you are sure to hit it."

Famously, Antoine de Saint-Exupery noted, "A goal without a plan is just a *wish.*"

Since college days, two poems have inspired me to set goals. They've recharged my inner batteries scores of times:

I shot my arrow into the sky.
It hit nothing. How it did fly.
I hit nothing for I did not try.
I just shot my arrow into the sky.
—Author unknown

Spring is past,
Summer is gone,
Winter is here,
And my song that I was meant to sing,
Is still unsung.
I have spent my days
Stringing and unstringing my
        instrument.
—Author unknown

In spite of adversities, the Boy Scout motto, "Always be prepared," has stood the test of time for me. Innumerable Navy SEALS, U. S. Rangers, military and corporate leaders, police, and others have benefitted from the Scout motto as well.

As a result of my scout training, I've done planning for vacations, workouts, book writing, speaking engagements, testy situations, and other settings. Of course, things haven't always gone the ways I wanted or planned.

I've read dozens of books on management, time-use, and planning. Most were worthwhile. One short book that helped me plan for possible future crises was Mary Ellen Copeland's, *WRAP: Wellness Action Recovery Plan*. It's loaded with practical tools and strategies for difficult challenges, especially addictions.

As a suggested step, write a one-page coping plan to use for your next possible hope-crisis. Share it with trusted friends or your professional healthcare provider. Then ask for their ideas.

QUESTIONS TO PONDER:

- How about taking a few minutes to write a one- or two-page plan for handling your next unfulfilled-dream crisis?
- With whom can you discuss it?

III

NAVIGATE YOUR
RELATIONSHIPS CAREFULLY

12

GET SUPPORT FROM OTHERS

*Two are better than one, because they have a good return for
their labor: If either of them falls down, one can help the other
up. But pity anyone who falls and has no one to help.*
—Ecclesiastes 4:9–10

It's painful to go through your bewildering loss alone.
Work at connecting regularly with friends who can
support and guide you. Attending a support group could
pay off well for you.

Probably the first step in letting go of an unrealistic wish is
to put your wished-for hopes clearly into words. Write
about your recent setback. Include your thoughts and feelings about your dented expectations. Then share your
writings with a safe friend, a clergy person, or a therapist.
Ask for their input in developing a healthy response for
relating to your offenders, or even help in confronting

them. The Bible teaches, *"Let the discerning get guidance. Make plans by seeking advice. Plans fail for lack of counsel, but with many advisers they succeed."*[1]

There are numerous studies confirming the value of quality relationships—for mental and physical well-being as well as extended longevity. While I tend to be a loner, I know that for my well-being I need other people. Knowing this, I work at developing and keeping supportive relationships. I encourage you to reach out and build your own support system. It will definitely pay off for you.

My most important relationship is with Leah, my wife. Since our early days of marriage, we've tried to share our highs and lows of each day and how we felt about them. Sure, we've occasionally missed days, but it has been a great way to log in with each other.

For nearly twenty years, I met weekly with several 12-step groups. The past two years I've met each week with a retired Marine friend and my men's sharing group. I also check in regularly with my special friend, Bob Long, by long-distance phone calls, texts, and emails. We also vacation together once a year or more.

QUESTIONS TO PONDER:

- Who do you have to lean on?
- Who depends on you?

13

GO WHERE THE LOVE IS, NOT WHERE IT SHOULD BE OR OUGHT TO BE

It took me way too long to realize that you shouldn't be friends with people who never ask how you are doing.
—Steve Maraboli

Hang around people and social events where love *is* rather than where it *should be*. This will help you minimize having your hopes repeatedly crushed. Suzy Kassem notes, "Spend your time with those who love you unconditionally, not those who love you *only* under certain conditions."

If possible, completely avoid—or, at the very least, lessen — your exposure to poisonous people, gatherings, and meetings. Michael Bessey Johnson warns:

> Stay away from lazy parasites, who perch on you just to satisfy their needs. They don't come to alleviate your burdens, hence, their mission is to distract, detract, and make you live in abject poverty.

Interestingly, the Apostle Paul gives notice of toxic gatherings: ". . . *your meetings do more harm than good.*"[1]

These "meetings" can easily refer to potentially harmful relationships with:

- *People*—your spouse, children, parents, siblings, relatives, neighbors, or other individuals such as your boss, co-worker, a company representative, or someone else who might do you emotional harm
- *Social Get-Togethers*—church meetings, social get-togethers, or community events

For example, George attended a Bible study support group meeting of thirty men and women. Most didn't have his social skills or Bible knowledge, and he was instrumental in helping others understand and apply what they were studying. The group facilitators often affirmed him for his contributions to the discussions; however, their accolades were so feeble, so hollow, they amounted to no compliment at all—damning him with faint praise.

It seemed to George that he was living out some of the zinging words of Alexander Pope's poetic satire, *Epistle to Dr. Arbuthnot:*

> Damn with faint praise, assent with
>   civil leer
> And, without sneering, teach the rest
>   to sneer;
> Willing to wound, and yet afraid to
>   strike,

> Just hint at a fault, and hesitate
> dislike.

Usually after others in the group shared, everyone applauded. Yet whenever George shared an insight, his words were met with deafening silence from the group.

Similar reactions by the leaders and group members continued every week. Each time he returned home feeling hurt, rejected, judged, resentful, and full of self-pity. At last, following a meeting two months ago, George sank into a depression that immobilized him. He cancelled three work days so he could recuperate from his having been slighted.

After those upsetting meetings, George concluded his presence evoked some kind of threat to the group and its leaders. Dejectedly, he felt his being there and offering comments were like "casting his pearls before swine." These people were probably jealous or simply unable to express appreciation to anyone.

Finally, he decided to stop absorbing any more unintentional or intentional hurts from the group. He simply quit and sought out another Bible study group.

Nevertheless, the leaders left him carrying a load of guilt, continuing to ask him why he'd dropped out. Without a clue for his withdrawal, they persisted in inviting him, "George, you have so much to offer the group. Why have you left us? We need you. How can you go elsewhere?

Centuries ago, the Bible advised, "It is to a man's honor to avoid strife. . . . A prudent man sees danger and takes refuge, but the simple keep going and suffer for it."[2]

George chose to keep away from being hurt again and again by his Bible group. He stopped attending and went instead to a different Bible study in his city.

QUESTIONS TO PONDER:

- Are you still returning to the same poisonous people, hoping you'll find your hopes restored?
- What can you do to protect yourself from another disillusionment?

14

DON'T RISK ILL-TIMED CONFRONTATIONS

Timing is everything. Therefore, you must discern when to make the most of each opportunity.
—Joy Marino

Not all confrontations are bad. Some are necessary. Usually they're stressful. Timing is crucial when confronting your expectations of someone or something. The Bible provides good sense on timing: *"There is a time for everything . . . a time to be silent and a time to speak."*[1]

Whenever you can, sidestep a setting or person who is poisonous—or even *might* be toxic. If necessary, lie low, hole up, and isolate for a while. Don't put yourself at risk for a big fall. Keep away from any person or circumstance that can possibly let you down. The Bible warns, *"So, if you think you are standing firm, be careful that you don't fall."*[2]

Even though I knew of the dangers, I risked attending some meetings, social gatherings, and meals with toxic persons. I rolled the dice chancing I wouldn't be mauled in some way with verbal disparagements.

Unfortunately, in gambling with touchy situations, I took some major hits. Those blows sometimes cost me days to recuperate from my inner hurt. Plus, I underwent relentless anxiety that future get-togethers would only repeat my wounds.

I recommend not taking chances on stepping into potentially risky circumstances with people, meetings, or social gatherings, even if you can win most of the time. If possible, play it safe. Avoid any adverse venue until you're less fragile.

QUESTIONS TO PONDER:

- Can you recall a poorly-timed confrontation you made?
- How did you feel after it blew up?
- What would you do differently if you could replay the scene?
- What lessons have you learned about confrontations?

15

DON'T TAKE PERSONALLY THE WORDS AND ACTIONS OF INSENSITIVE PEOPLE

If you take everything personally and to heart, it will tear you apart. Take criticism, learn, adjust, and move on.
—Johnny Iuzzini

I've discovered that stewing over offenses or retaliating for others' motives is usually a wasted effort. Much of the time, trying to figure out what you might have said or done to trigger a negative comment is a useless exercise that leads only to frustration.

The same fruitless results happen when you spend hours searching for the reason for your offender's behavior.

Even though he was a remarkable follower of Christ, the Apostle Paul suffered heartbreaking hope-losses— when some trusted friends deserted him:

You know that everyone in the Province of Asia has deserted me, including Phygelus and Hermogenes. . . . Demas, because he loved this world, has deserted me and has gone to Thessolonica.

—2 Timothy 1:15; 4:10

Alas, both Christians and non-believers can act in deceitful or harmful ways. I've found that about 90% of the lies, put downs, betrayals, and broken promises I've endured have little or nothing to do with *me*.

My advisors suggested that I look at my wrongdoers' track records of relationships. It shocked me to discover that I wasn't alone in being injured by untrustworthy people. I noticed my tormentors had exhibited *similar* patterns of behaviors toward others: lies, deceits, misrepresentations, broken agreements, put downs, defamations, and slanderous comments. I was only one on a long list of victims.

I also noticed that stresses in my persecutors' lives were intensifying their actions. There was nothing I had done wrong. They were simply reacting to pain in their own lives—taking it out on me and others.

Sometimes I've observed that both Christian and non-Christian promise-breakers have some kind of psychological need to feel better about themselves by pulling others down or causing them to stumble in some way. The wrongdoers were simply liars and schemers who did or said whatever it took to make themselves look good, even at someone else's expense.

Laurie Notaro discerns, "If you really believe in what you're doing, work hard, take nothing personally and if something blocks one route, find another. Never give up." My newly learned lesson: don't always take everything personally.

Many of my former "friends" had been unresponsive to all my attempts to communicate. My counselors suggested that I should give up trying to rebuild bridges with these unresponsive individuals. I took their advice and ended my hope of resuming old "friendships."

As a result of their counsel, I stopped asking my ex-friends to get together for coffee or lunch, texting, emailing, or phoning. In the place of those severed relationships, I strengthened my current and old friendships.

QUESTIONS TO PONDER:

- Have you shared with someone else your self-blame for your friends' behaviors?
- What will it take for you to cease trying to re-establish a long-time broken relationship?

IV

DRAW ON SPIRITUAL
SOURCES FOR STRENGTH

16

RELEASE CONTROL OF YOUR CIRCUMSTANCES TO GOD

Find rest, O my soul, in God alone; my hope comes from him. He alone is my mighty rock . . . my fortress . . . Trust in him at all times, O people; pour out your hearts to him, for God is our refuge.
—Psalm 62:5–8

Here's a suggestion from me and fellow dream-gutted fighters: even though you might not be an alcoholic, practice applying the first three revised steps of *Alcoholics Anonymous* to your ruined expectations.

1. Admit you are powerless over your lost hopes and that your reactions to your losses have become unmanageable.
2. Come to believe that a Power greater than yourself can restore you to balanced thinking about your loss.

3. Make a decision to turn your will and your life over to the care of God as you understand Him.

I applied these steps to my circumstances. First, I started by admitting to myself that that my life had become unmanageable and that I was powerless over being upset by my quashed plans. I acknowledged that I couldn't control either the outcome of my conditions or my unhealthy responses to them. I conceded that all my efforts to remain calm had failed.

Second, I resigned my own dismal attempts to solve the problem and admitted to myself that only God could restore me to healthy emotional balance.

Third, I reflected on the phrase: "I can't, but God can, so I'll let him." I surrendered to God's management of my anxieties of living without my vision's fruition. Then I made a purposeful decision to turn my will, my life with all its disrupted hopes, and my future over to God's care, protection, and guidance. Implementing those three steps of AA gained me more balanced thinking and inner peace.

QUESTIONS TO PONDER:

- Have you admitted to yourself that you are unable to resurrect your hope, and that you are having unhealthy reactions to your loss?
- Have you come to the place where you believe that only God can help you?
- Are you willing to let go and let God take charge of either rescuing your dream or changing it?

17

KEEP ASKING GOD FOR HIS HELP AND GUIDANCE

You hear, O Lord, the desire of the afflicted; you encourage them,
and you listen to their cry.
—Psalm 10:17

Innumerable times I and countless others have been sustained by words from the Christian Scriptures, and by calling out to God in our confusion for his help. I know I wouldn't have made it through my many letdowns without God's reassurance, energizing, and guidance. The Bible explains God's special guidance for his people as they plan new hopes:

The Lord will guide you always; He will satisfy your needs in a
sun-scorched land and will strengthen your frame.

—Isaiah 49:10

I will lead the blind by ways they have not known, along
unfamiliar paths I will guide them; I will turn the darkness into

light before them and make the rough places smooth. These are the things I will do; I will not forsake them.

—Isaiah 42:16

Forget the former things; do not dwell on the past. See, I am doing a new thing! Now it springs up; do you not perceive it? I am making a way in the desert and streams in the wasteland.

—Isaiah 43:18, 19

Saying the well-known *Serenity Prayer*, attributed to Reinhold Niebuhr (1892–1971), can give you fresh perspective and better resilience—to lower, raise, or let go of your anxieties and expectations. Try praying the *Serenity Prayer* whenever you feel stressed:

God, grant me the serenity to accept the things I cannot change; courage to change the things I can; and wisdom to know the difference. Living one day at a time; enjoying one moment at a time; accepting hardship as the pathway to peace; taking, as He did, this sinful world as it is, not as I would have it; trusting that He will make all things right if I surrender to His will; that I may be reasonably happy in this life, and supremely happy with Him forever in the next. Amen.

Thousands of others can join me in testify to the life-changing help that comes from praying and putting into practice the *Serenity Prayer*. If you haven't tried it, why not experiment by employing the *Serenity Prayer* yourself?

QUESTIONS TO PONDER:

- What have you got to lose by reaching out to God with your honest doubts, hurts, or crumpled hopes?
- What reassurances do you need from him?
- What guidance do you need from him?

18

THANK GOD EACH MORNING FOR THREE BLESSINGS YOU RECEIVED YESTERDAY

Praise the Lord, O my soul, and forget not all his benefits. . . I will sing to the Lord for he has been good to me. . . in the morning I will sing of your love.
—Psalm 103:2, 13:6, 59:16

It's so easy to concentrate on our missing hope and our life without it, but rehashing a failed anticipation merely churns up undesirable emotions.

Expressing gratitude doesn't deny life's difficulties, nor does it fix problems, but a thankful heart opens us up to countless good things. Giving thanks will help you start your day with an upbeat outlook.

Here are two workable suggestions that can help you become more thankful in the midst of heartache:

1. Throughout the day, try to voice your appreciation

to God or other people for something good they did for you. Practice this not only in good times, but also when you become aware of a resentment, no matter how petty it may seem.

2. Try keeping a "Gratitude Journal." Jotting down daily instances of God's intervening help can change your perspective on everything. Some people find this practice extremely helpful. However, I've not been disciplined enough to do this for any length of time. For me, simply voicing my gratitude to God every morning has been enough to make a difference.

Several years ago, at a 12-step meeting, someone mentioned the importance of giving thanks daily for three of God's blessings of the previous day. I've followed this recommendation nearly every day for twenty-five years. And this simple habit has done wonders for my outlook.

Yes, there have been times when my whole world collapsed on me shortly after my thanking God, but the benefits of giving thanks are exceedingly helpful. Even when my life snags on obstacles, I've found my daily praise keeps me connected to God in the midst of bad storms.

Andrea and Michael enjoyed a forty-eight-year marriage. They looked forward to their next year's retirement, with plans to travel, take up new hobbies, and spend more time with their children and grandchildren.

Suddenly, during his yearly physical, the routine tests showed that Michael had a terminal brain tumor. His doctors gave him less than one month to live.

In a moment, all their looked-forward-to plans were wiped out—replaced by escalating fears, doctor's appointments, and cancelled trips.

Hard, gut-wrenching times followed. Nevertheless, in the midst of their foreboding anxiety, Andrea and Michael started thanking God each morning for the blessings of the day before.

What a difference expressing gratitude to God made in their attitudes. Rather than being overcome by fears, their new routine of giving thanks to God daily enabled them to adapt to their bleak reality. They appreciated much more the time together they had left.

QUESTIONS TO PONDER:

- How will you spend your solitary conversations with yourself today—by listing your complaints or by counting your blessings?
- What difference will expressing gratefulness mean to you and your circumstances?
- How about trying a three-week tryout of thanking God each morning for his blessings of yesterday?

V

MAINTAIN THE RIGHT MINDSET

19

ALLOW YOURSELF TO GRIEVE*

None of us are immune to grief, and everyone who has suffered loss understands that grief changes, but you never wake up one morning and you've moved on. It stays with you; and, you know, you ebb and flow.
—Terri Irwin

Letting go of coveted yearnings that aren't being fulfilled is a mourning process, and despair is a necessary step. This deep sadness can be agonizingly painful, but it won't last forever.

Here are a few thoughts compiled by a panel of grief therapists on grieving your missing hope:

- Grieving isn't a sign of weakness; it's a sign that you are being honest about the feelings in your heart.

- It's okay to tell family and friends how you feel and what you want them to do to help you go through the passing away of your longed-for dream.
- Don't suppress the pain you feel; it will only resurface later. Experience it, feel it, and resist the temptation to stuff it away or numb its pain with harmful behaviors or substance abuses.
- Seek out people who understand what you are experiencing. Perhaps join a grief support group or see a grief counselor.
- Talk with God, no matter how you feel. Even if you are angry, tell God. He's big enough to handle your pain and your questions.

I grieved for my lost hopes of recumbent bicycle-riding, the hurt of "friends" who'd abandoned me, and hurts by noxious people. By sharing my pain, I found a peace that calmed my upsets. My wife, close friends, my men's sharing group, and my therapist became a powerful support system.

As I *faced* the absence of my vanished hopes, I was able to mourn. I learned that grieving my losses was vital for my healing and growth. Strangely, my sorrow brought added perspective, fresh ideas, new hopes. As I lamented, I let go of my long-awaited wishes that *couldn't* be. In letting go, I freed my energies to invest in hopes that *could* be.

QUESTIONS TO PONDER:

- Have you given yourself permission to feel deep sadness for the demise of your dream?
- What people can you safely disclose your loss-reactions with, without being lectured or judged?

20

DISTRACT YOURSELF FROM NEGATIVE THINKING

Time doesn't heal emotional pain;
you need to learn to let it go.
—Roy T. Benett

It's easy to sit and stew about the unfairness of it all, but a boiling bitterness toward someone or something can sour your outlook and spoil your relationships.

In your crisis, it will help to do *anything* that can distract you from "stinking thinking."

Diverting your negative thoughts can take your mind off your recent distress, as well as the anxiety over the dread of going on without your hoped-for expectation. Timely actions can keep your obsessive thoughts at bay. Experiment with these or other activities until you find what works for you:

- practice a hobby
- sleep
- read
- listen to music
- watch TV, videos, or a movie
- take a walk
- enjoy a sports event
- do something to help someone
- get a massage

I've used all of these tools at various times to redirect my mental replays from obsessing over my absent hopes to positive matters. Yet, sometimes what works well in one situation will fail in another, so I experimented with different ways to escape my negative thinking.

Richard, my neighbor, wasn't able to deflect his self-defeating thoughts. He was a heartbroken father who strongly anticipated having a close relationship with his son, but by tenth grade Richard's hopes were dashed by his son's mental illness and drug-addiction.

Richard replayed his thwarted longings over and over, unwilling to shake off his destructive thinking. He buried the pain of his missing father/son bond by working longer hours at a frenzied pace. When the reality of his caved-in dreams finally sunk in, Richard collapsed emotionally. A week later he was hospitalized for suicidal depression.

QUESTIONS TO PONDER:

- What tactics are you willing to experiment with to

free yourself from painful reminders of your missing hope?

- What steps can you take to avoid potential consequences of "stinking thinking" like Richard faced?
- What's holding you back from experimenting with various escape tools?

21

DO SOMETHING EVERY DAY TO
TREAT YOURSELF

Self-love, my liege, is not so vile a sin as self-neglecting.
—William Shakespeare

Persevering through the trauma of a battered hope requires special self-care. Stifled hopes drain energy, warp attitudes, and devolve into neglecting your own needs. Maybe this is why Jesus's second greatest commandment is to "*Love your neighbor as yourself.*"[1]

Healthy self-love is extremely important. When your expectations have been sidetracked, it's easy to become consumed with self-condemnation, self-absorbed misery, paranoia, cynicism, or mistrust of people. Doing positive things for yourself and others can be a powerful antidote for destructive negativity.

I seem to function best with my responsibilities when I, like a donkey, have a carrot held out in front of me—a reward of some kind: a movie to see, a new piece of exercise equipment to use, a trip to the mountains, or some other incentive for my efforts.

Why not try a special indulgence for yourself with a:

- hobby,
- bubble bath,
- massage,
- sports event,
- concert,
- tasty meal, or
- gift just for yourself.

If you can't or don't want to nurture yourself, you can take happiness to *others*. There may be times when you cannot take good care of yourself due to depression, self-loathing, agitation, or some other malady.

When this is the case, try to shift from caring for yourself to meeting the needs of others. Believe it or not, helping others can bless both the you and your recipient. This is one reason the Bible also teaches, "Blessed is he who is kind to the needy."[2]

Actor Will Smith affirms, "Helping *others* with encouraging words or practical assistance will not only benefit them, but will also be especially gratifying for you.

If you're not making someone else's life better, then you're wasting your time. Your life will become better by making other lives better."

If you're having trouble caring for your own needs, why not reach out to *someone else in need* with a:

- word of encouragement;
- note, text, or email offering your support;
- small gift;
- volunteering to use your time, skills, or tools— babysitting, fixing an appliance, raking leaves, repairing a car, helping with computer advice, or some other service;
- prayer with and for them; or
- phone call inviting someone for coffee or lunch.

This is what Sandy did. She is a fifty-five-year-old wife and mother of three who sobbed recounting how her husband of thirty-one years had recently left her for another woman.

Her hopes of retirement with him were gone. In the wake of her loss, Sandy battled one health issue after another, including frequent panic attacks.

To cope with her worst times, Sandy did two things:

First, on her really bad days when reminders of her husband's betrayal hit her the hardest, she took several "mental health days" to comfort her wounded spirit. She slept in, treated herself to a much-loved pasta meal, watched her favorite TV shows, or soaked in hot bubble baths.

Second, Sandy reached out to two other recently divorced, financially strapped women. She invited them to go to a concert with her, giving them a luxury they wouldn't have been able to afford on their own. Doing this "good deed" helped take her mind off her own pain.

QUESTIONS TO PONDER:

- What "carrots" appeal to you as encouragements while you muddle through your damaged dream?
- How can you boost someone else's concerns with some kind of caring encouragement?

22

REMIND YOURSELF OFTEN THAT "THIS TOO SHALL PASS"

A person is about as happy as he makes up his mind to be.
—Abraham Lincoln

Years ago, after I had to fire a popular church employee, many members were angry with me for months. Their upset was reflected in their constant opposition to any plans I initiated. They halted their financial giving and recruited others to stir up other members to oppose me. The turmoil took its toll. Every day my insides churned.

I certainly could identify with the words of Olympic running star, Jesse Owens: "The battles that count aren't the ones for gold medals. The struggles within yourself—the invisible, inevitable battles inside all of us—that's where it's at."

I could see no end of resistance to my leadership at that church, only escalating opposition. The hard but simple way out of my dismal attitude was to discuss the matter with some close friends and remind myself continually, "This too will pass." It took a long time, but eventually the problem worked itself out.

Sometimes it was helpful to think thoughts like:

- What difference will this difficulty make in ten years?
- Life will certainly bring other trials for me to face, so I might as well practice handling this painful situation.
- It will benefit me in the long run if I shoulder these latest wounds and not indulge in feeling victimized or seek some kind of revenge.

In some situations, saying out loud some of *Alcoholics Anonymous'* mottos have gotten me through a host of difficulties:

- "Think."
- "First things first."
- "Easy does it."
- "Keep it simple."
- "One day at a time."
- "Listen and learn."
- "Let go and let God."

In the same way, several U.S. Navy SEAL slogans have pushed me forward on innumerable occasions:

- "The only easy day was yesterday."

- "Get comfortable with being uncomfortable."
- "Embrace the suck."
- "No plan survives first contact with the enemy."

In similar fashion, successful athletes, special ops soldiers, business leaders, and thousands of others use differing slogans to keep themselves on an even keel during precarious moments. Some invent their own mantras; others repeat well-known ones.

QUESTIONS TO PONDER:

- What slogans can you use to reinforce your resolve?
- What tactics are you willing to experiment with to free yourself from painful reminders of your missing hope?
- Do you have anyone who can encourage you during your tough times?

23

TAKE PERSONAL RESPONSIBILITY FOR YOUR REACTIONS TO DISRUPTED HOPES

When one door of happiness closes, another opens; but often we look so long at the closed door that we do not see the one which has been opened for us.
—Helen Keller

Dr. Robert Schuller offers this valuable counsel, "If it's going to be, it's up to *me*." This advice goes for either manipulating dreams to materialize, altering certain goals, or aborting specific plans.

It's important to decide *how* you want to handle your smashed expectations. Do you want to continue to have your hope dashed again and again? Do you want to go on using up your time to pursue your dream? Do you want to spend your energies fixating on injustices dealt to you or on developing new hopes?

Once you face the fact that you are being triggered by negatives, admit to yourself that unless you *do* something to check their influence, your damaging reactions have the power to cause internal hurts that can devastate you and all whom you care about.

It's critical to own up to the certainty that your thoughts and emotions over your loss make you vulnerable to being harmed in the future. You, like many who've had optimisms burst, are at risk for unraveling emotionally and spiritually. If not dealt with, this flawed sense of self-sufficiency can lead you to a dangerous relapse of ruined relationships, severe agitations, or a deep depression.

The Apostle Paul was constantly troubled by a "thorn in his flesh." He could have considered his thorn issue a failure and been immobilized by his difficulty. Instead, he took action. While he continued to pray for God to remove his obstacle, Paul kept making tents and preaching.

Yet, God told him to stop praying about the thorn because it would not be removed. So Paul gave up on his wish for a thorn-free life and chose to invest his energies on other things like writing, teaching, and encouraging others.

My younger brother, Bob, an experienced marathon runner, died suddenly from a blood clot in 2003. I, also, had two clots after two surgeries a decade ago. In 2018, after being hospitalized for a blood clot behind my left knee, my doctors put me on a blood thinner to prevent future clots.

Being on a blood thinner also carries high risks for excessive bleeding. A crash on my recumbent bike could be life threatening. I discussed my options with my doctors. The answer was clear: the risks of falling and bleeding were too great. No more bike riding.

I could have done nothing and continued to ride, waiting for a new miracle drug or for God to heal me, but I decided to be proactive. I contacted the *Semper Fi Marine Fund* at Camp Pendleton, California, and donated my expensive bike and equipment to a wounded Marine.

I didn't wait for God or others to somehow bail me out of my wrecked plans for resuming my recumbent bike rides. Instead, I assumed personal responsibility for keeping a positive attitude following my loss.

For me, taking charge of my own "healing" involved reading on recovery methods, writing about my smashed hopes, talking about my plight with supportive friends, and getting counseling from my therapist.

Recently, I was challenged by a sign written by a sage thinker:

> You've got three choices in life:
> give up,
> give in, or
> give it all you've got.

I've trudged through all three of these options as I've processed my many vaporized hopes. I'm so grateful that God and others helped me to take responsibility and give it my all—moving ahead despite my losses. Writing this book is one of my choices to move ahead with my life instead of smoldering with resentment over the hopes that are nowhere to be found.

QUESTIONS TO PONDER:

- Are you still waiting for someone or something to happen that will solve your vanished hope?
- What will it take for *you* to now take charge of recovering from the hurt, resentment, or bitterness of missing your long-hoped-for dream?

FIND RESOURCES FOR COPING AND REBUILDING

Whatever is true, whatever is noble, whatever is right, whatever is admirable — if anything is excellent or praiseworthy — think about such things.
—Philippians 4:8

Recovery resources are basic to your well-being during and following a major loss. Sometimes, you'll come across resources *in the midst* of your trauma that help you to keep going, but, *after* your trauma you'll want *other* life-enhancing resources to go forward with your rebuilding.

Your resources could be:

- positive people who affirm you and are pleasant to be around;
- inspirational literature such as the Bible, self-help information, websites, and others;

- biographies;
- novels;
- jokes;
- music;
- movies or videos; or
- concerts.

These or other aids can foster a healthy rebounding from your crushed hope.

Reading on recovery from trauma or talking with crushed-hope alumnae will give you fresh viewpoints on recovering from your inner injuries. Your conversations can result in huge paybacks. These sources can enrich your healing from hurts.

The Bible has played a central role in my dealing with annihilated expectations. Several other books were also valuable in keeping me afloat as I mended from mangled possibilities. During some of my worst periods, jokes and self-help literature have lifted me up from my despair.

Strangely, joking often provided me with a welcome perspective on upsets. The author of Proverbs describes the value of humor: *"He who is of a merry heart has a continual feast . . . A merry heart does good, like medicine."* [1]

For recurring hope-disappointments, I found Carey Nieuwhof 's book, *Didn't See It Coming: Overcoming the 7 Greatest Challenges That No One Expects* particularly useful. Two other books provided me with much needed courage to persevere: Lewis Smedes's book, *Keeping Hope Alive: For a Tomorrow We Cannot Control* and H. Norman Wright's, *Resilience: Rebounding When Life's Upsets Knock You Down.*

QUESTIONS TO PONDER:

- What gives you the most energy to continue?
- What personal resources have helped you to hold on, even when life has been most challenging?
- What new motivational actions would you like to try?

REVIEWING KEY POINTS

To review how you can overcome your crushed hopes and unmet expectations, here are the 24 suggested guidelines we've discussed:

1. Accept the reality of your lost hopes.
2. Count the cost of pursuing your fading dream— for you and others.
3. Let go of your aspirations for yourself, other people, or situations.
4. Let go of your hurt, anger, and desire for revenge.
5. Don't secretly cling to your expectations.
6. Take a mental inventory of your letdowns.
7. If you often have unrealistic expectations, lower your expectation bar.
8. In certain cases, try raising your expectation bar.
9. Go with the solution that works, not one that should work.
10. Revise your past goals or set new ones.
11. Plan ahead for future, unmet expectations.

12. Get support from others.
13. Go where the love is, not where it should be or ought to be.
14. Don't risk ill-timed confrontations.
15. Don't take personally the words and actions of insensitive people.
16. Release control of your circumstances to God.
17. Keep asking God for his help and guidance.
18. Thank God each morning for three blessings you received yesterday.
19. Allow yourself to grieve.
20. Distract yourself from negative thinking.
21. Do something every day to treat yourself.
22. Remind yourself often that "This too shall pass."
23. Take personal responsibility for your reactions to disrupted hopes.
24. Find resources for coping and rebuilding.

CONCLUSION

Micah Herndon is a thirty-one-year-old U.S. Marine veteran who served in Iraq and Afghanistan. He survived an IED explosion and now deals with severe PTSD. His running helps to keep the side-effects at bay. On April 15, 2019, Micah ran the 26.2-mile Boston Marathon—to honor his fallen comrades and to qualify for running in the upcoming New York City Marathon with a qualifying time of three hours, thirteen minutes.

About 4.2 miles before the end of the race, both his legs cramped and seized up. In order to achieve his Boston Marathon dream, he dragged himself at a slow, power-walk pace. With nearly 100 yards to go, he could no longer move his legs.

So he crawled on his hands and knees to cross the finish line in an incredible 3 hours and 38 minutes! Not good enough time to be eligible for the New York run, but finishing the race resulted in great honor for his soldier friends.

Micah's hoped-for dream of *running* the whole marathon had been wiped out. He could have quit when his dream ended, but he switched hopes. Instead of dropping out of the marathon because he could no longer run the full race, he slowly *inched* on his knees those nearly 100 yards.

The next day Micah was interviewed on the *Today* Show. Asked how he gutted out the final 100 yards on his knees, he simply said, "It was the longest 4.2 miles I've ever run in my life, but I'm a Marine. Our slogan is, 'Adapt and survive'."

It wasn't easy for Micah, me, and others who've overcome our damaged hopes. Some of us have had to rework, change, drop, or create new hopes. For me, it usually felt like I was taking second best. Yet what else could I do?

What else can *you* do about your evaporated dreams? Most likely, making a hope substitution won't be a stress free, uncomplicated, or painless task for you, but the rewards will be well-worth the effort.

My sincere desire for you, my reader, is that God will enable you to hang onto your unmet hopes, or that you'll adapt to the reality that they will never come back—by accepting your loss, changing your expectation or discovering a new hoped-for wish.

ACKNOWLEDGMENTS

Rarely, if ever, does a book become published without an enormous *team* effort. This book is no exception. I am grateful to the following people of my "writing team," without whom this book would not have been completed:

- Bob Long, Cliff Ishigaki, Jake Swartout, Bob Johnson, Paul Tennyson, Randy Speer, Steve Allee, and Ken Kroeger who, time and time again, listened, gave feedback, and shared timely jokes to help me bounce back after unexpected or long-lasting hindrances.
- Dr. Laurel Basbas and Dr. Himasiri De Silva, my psychologist and psychiatrist, whose professional expertise and encouragement kept me going after a variety of setbacks.
- Andrew Kroeger, my brilliant editor, whose skills, insights, and dedicated work made such a huge difference in sculpting these pages.
- Elijah Dove, my copyeditor, and Eldrid Hinton

and Frank Canin, my proofreaders, whose talents corrected grammar and typing errors and honed this manuscript.

- Maggie Dillon, my computer "techie" and typist, who input numerous quotes and manuscript changes, and kept me from pulling out my hair over so many electronic glitches.
- Stephanie Reese, my dedicated office manager, whose clerical and organizational abilities supplied countless hours of copying and collating of research articles and enabled me to focus on writing.
- Ellen Enochs, my loyal friend, whose support and cheerleading actions boosted my spirits time and again.
- Above all, I am most thankful for Leah, my wife of 50+ years, who sacrificed many of our togetherness times and helped me to stay the writing course for this and other books. Her never-ending reassurance inspired me to keep going through one crushed hope after another.

Thank you, special team!

NOTES

INTRODUCTION

1. Proverbs 13:19, emphasis added
2. Hebrews 12:15
3. Acts 8:23

4. LET GO OF YOUR HURT, ANGER, AND DESIRE FOR REVENGE

1. Proverbs 20:22

10. REVISE YOUR PAST GOALS OR SET NEW ONES

1. Jeremiah 29:11

11. PLAN AHEAD FOR FUTURE, UNMET EXPECTATIONS

1. Proverbs 14:8; 22:3

12. GET SUPPORT FROM OTHERS

1. Proverbs 1:5, 20:18, 15:22

13. GO WHERE THE LOVE IS, NOT WHERE IT SHOULD BE OR OUGHT TO BE

1. 1 Cor.11:17
2. Proverbs 20:3, 22:3

14. DON'T RISK ILL-TIMED CONFRONTATIONS

1. Ecclesiastes 3:1, 7
2. 1 Corinthians 10:12

21. DO SOMETHING EVERY DAY TO TREAT YOURSELF

1. Mark 12:31, emphasis added
2. Proverbs 14:21

24. FIND RESOURCES FOR COPING AND REBUILDING

1. Proverbs 15:15; 17:22

CAN YOU HELP ME WITH SOMETHING?

Thank you for reading this book. I hope you've been encouraged by it! If you've found it especially helpful and worthy of a recommendation, can you help me with something?

Will you please email me with a couple of sentences as a mini book review? You could share what you liked about the book and how it impacted your life. Potential readers will be encouraged by your words!

WANT TO STAY UP TO DATE WITH MY NEW BOOKS AND ARTICLES?

Subscribe to my newsletter for great articles, behind-the-scenes looks at upcoming books, and a FREE digital copy of my book *9 Critical Steps to take in a Mental Health Crisis*.

Visit www.drjimstout.com/join to subscribe.

Dr. Stout has been a pastor, leader, husband, and loving father, yet in the past he's also been clinically depressed and suicidal. His easy-to-read books describe his experiences and recovery. They share the techniques he and others have used to heal themselves, and offer tools to reclaim your life and move forward!

All books are (or soon will be) available online through Amazon. Further information can be found by visiting Dr. Stout's website at www.drjimstout.com.

Please consider purchasing some of these life-enhancing publications for yourself, or as gifts for family members, friends, patients, clergy, and mental and medical health providers. They are ideal for encouragement gifts, bulk orders, special promotions, and other uses.

A portion of the profits from these books will be used to support four ministries: wounded veterans, mentally ill patients and families, career guidance, and clergy counseling.

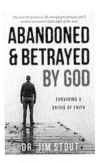

Discover the practical, life-changing techniques you'll need to overcome a dark night of the soul.

ABANDONED & BETRAYED BY GOD

SURVIVING A CRISIS OF FAITH

DR. JIM STOUT

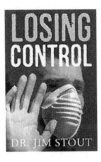

LOSING CONTROL

DR. JIM STOUT

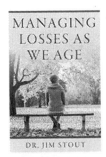

MANAGING LOSSES AS WE AGE

DR. JIM STOUT

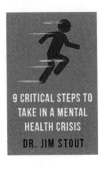

9 CRITICAL STEPS TO TAKE IN A MENTAL HEALTH CRISIS

DR. JIM STOUT

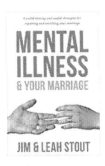

Candid, bracing and useful strategies for repairing and enriching your marriage

MENTAL ILLNESS
& YOUR MARRIAGE

JIM & LEAH STOUT

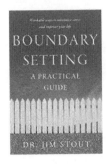

Workable ways to minimize stress and improve your life

BOUNDARY SETTING
A PRACTICAL GUIDE

DR. JIM STOUT

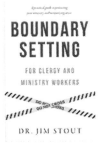

Expert tools & paths to protecting your sanctuary and sustaining joy at work

BOUNDARY SETTING

FOR CLERGY AND MINISTRY WORKERS

DO NOT CROSS
DO NOT CROSS

DR. JIM STOUT

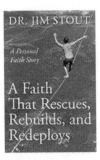

DR. JIM STOUT

A Personal Faith Story

A Faith That Rescues, Rebuilds, and Redeploys

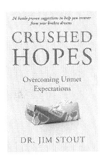

24 battle-proven suggestions to help you recover from your broken dreams

CRUSHED HOPES

Overcoming Unmet Expectations

DR. JIM STOUT

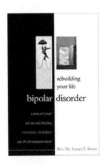

rebuilding your life

bipolar disorder

A BIPOLAR'S DIARY THAT INCLUDES PRACTICAL STRATEGIES FOR, STEP-BY-STEP, REBUILDING YOUR LIFE AND TIPS FOR REMAINING WELL

Rev. Dr. James T. Stout

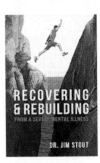

RECOVERING & REBUILDING

FROM A SEVERE MENTAL ILLNESS

DR. JIM STOUT

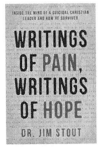

INSIDE THE MIND OF A SUICIDAL CHRISTIAN LEADER AND HOW HE SURVIVED

WRITINGS OF PAIN, WRITINGS OF HOPE

DR. JIM STOUT

ABOUT THE AUTHOR

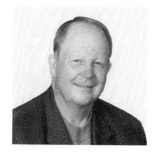 Rev. Dr. James T. Stout is an ordained Presbyterian pastor. He has ministered in five churches and volunteered in five others.

His other ministry experiences include working with college and graduate students at Harvard, MIT, Boston, Northeastern, and Miami universities; doing social work with Young Life's outreach to teenage gangs in New York City; being student chaplain to the men's violent ward at Danvers Massachusetts State Mental Hospital; serving as an area director with The Gathering USA, a national ministry with business and professional men; and founding Rebuilding Your Life, a career counseling service.

Dr. Stout has spoken to professional football and baseball chapels, business and professional leader groups, high school and college student classes, mental illness conferences, workshops and seminars, classes at Fuller and Gordon-Conwell seminaries, and numerous churches. He has also served on the advisory board for clinical pastoral education at the Crystal Cathedral in Garden Grove, California. Find out more by visiting www.drjimstout.com.

Made in the USA
Columbia, SC
27 November 2024

47201720R10081